Copyright - 2021 - All rights ed, The content contained within t duplicated, or transmitted wi ion from the author or the publish Under no circumstances will an be held against the publisher, or author, for any damages, reparation, or monetary loss due to the information contained within this book.
Either directly or indirectly.

Legal Notice:

This book is copyright protected. This book is only for personal use. You cannot amend, distribute, sell, use, quote, or paraphrase any part of the content within this book without the author or publisher's consent.

Disclaimer Notice:

Please note the information contained within this document is for educational and entertainment purposes only. All effort has been executed to present accurate, up-to-date, and reliable, complete information. No warranties of any kind are declared or implied.

Readers acknowledge that the author is not engaging in the rendering of legal, financial, medical, or professional advice. The content within this book has been derived from various sources. Please consult a licensed professional before attempting any techniques outlined in this book.

By reading this document, the reader agrees that under no circumstances is the author responsible for any losses, direct or indirect, which are incurred as a result of the use of the information contained within this document, including, but not limited to, - errors, omissions, or inaccuracies.

APPETIZERS AND SNACKS 5

LOBSTER SALAD IN ENDIVE	6
HOT ARTICHOKE AND SPINACH DIP	9
	11
GUACAMOLE DIP OR SALAD DRESSING	12
HOT CRAB DIP	15
CRAB-CHEESE DIP	17
TUNA DIP	18
CHICKEN CHEESE DIP	19
CHEESE PUFFS	20
STUFFED MOZZARELLA	22
ARTICHOKE-SPINACH DIP	24
FRESH CRAB COCKTAIL	25
CRAB COCKTAIL	27
CRABBIE SPREAD	28
CHEESE BALL	29
OPTIONS FOR CHIPS AND DIPPERS	31
CREAM CHEESE/BLEU CHEESE/PESTO	33
CHICKEN "PASTE"	34
BACON CHEDDAR DIP	36
TOASTED SEASONED NUTS	38
STUFFED MUSHROOMS	40
SPINACH DIP	42
GUACAMOLE	43
SALSA CHEESECAKE	46
CURRIED PUMPKIN SEEDS	49
SMOKED GOUDA-STUFFED CHICKEN WRAPPED IN BACON	51
BEEF COIN SNACKS	54
OYSTERS IN GRUYERE SAUCE	55

LOW-CARBOHYDRATE GUACAMOLE	56
TAPENADE	57
MOZZARELLA STICKS	59
FRIED VIETNAMESE SPRING ROLLS	62
HOMEMADE ANTIPASTO	66
MUSHROOM PATE	67
CRAB STUFFED MUSHROOMS	69
PICKLED SHRIMP	70
CRABMEAT DIP	73
SALMON DIP	74
CARBOHYDRATE-FREE NACHOS	76
SPINACH DIP	77
HOT CRAB DIP	79
PORTOBELLOS WITH FETA AND ARTICHOKES	80
SCALLOPS OR SHRIMP WITH BACON	81
LOW-CARB CHEESE STICKS	81
THAI SHRIMP DIP	83
MACADAMIA PESTO	86

BEVERAGES 88

CHOCOLATE SHAKE	89
HOT CHOCOLATE	90
FRAPPUCCINO	90
STRAWBERRY SHAKE	91
PROTEIN SHAKE	92
PROTEIN "MILKSHAKES"	93
QUICK PROTEIN SHAKE	94
HOT COCOA	95
COCONUTTY PROTEIN SHAKE	96

SHAKE SHAKE	97
PROTEIN SHAKE ALA LIGHT	98
FAVORITE PROTEIN SHAKE RECIPE	99
PROTEIN POWER SHAKE	100
THE FRUGAL GAZETTE DIET DRINK	101
PROTEIN SHAKE BASE WITH VARIATIONS	103
SHAKE RECIPE	105
"SPICE TEA" MIX	106
BREAKFAST ON THE GO	107
RASPBERRY PROTEIN SHAKE	107
HOT CHOCOLATE	108
"BAILEY'S AND COFFEE"	109
EGGNOG	109
EGG NOT	111

APPETIZERS AND SNACKS

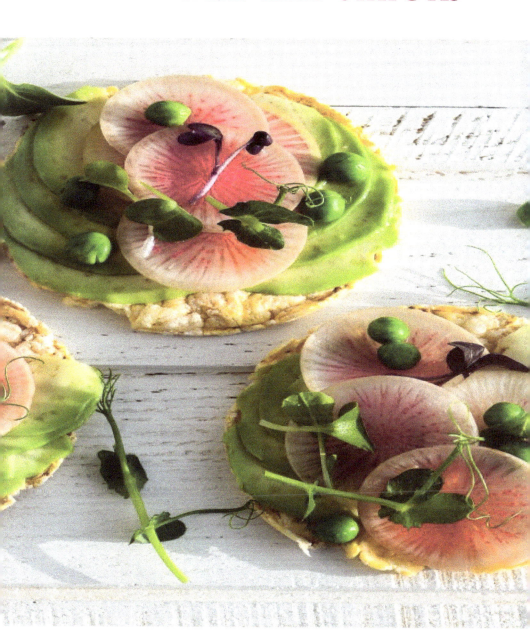

Lobster Salad in Endive

Makes 24 appetizers; serves 6 to 8

If you want to be good to yourself and your guests at the same time, ask your fish store to sell you cooked fresh lobster meat instead of cooking a lobster yourself. This is a great summer appetizer or a special treat for New Year's Eve. This recipe is also good, and not quite so expensive, with cooked shrimp or crabmeat. You'll see that a little salad makes a lot of appetizers.

Ingredients

- 3/4 pound freshly cooked lobster meat, small-diced
- 1/2 cup good mayonnaise
- 1/2 cup small-diced celery (1 stalk)
- 1 tablespoon capers, drained
- 1 1/2 tablespoons minced fresh dill Pinch kosher salt, pinch freshly ground black pepper
- 4 heads Belgian endive

Combine the lobster, mayonnaise, celery, capers, dill, salt, and pepper. With a sharp knife, cut off the base of the endive and separate the leaves. Use a teaspoon to fill the end of each endive leaf with lobster salad. Arrange on a platter and serve.

Make sure you use real lobster, though. I was perusing through my carbohydrate counter just yesterday at fish and seafood and noticed that the fake lobster or crab is really pretty high in carbohydrates at 8.5 carbs per 3 oz.

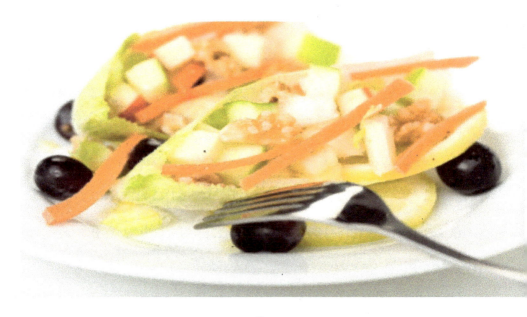

Hot Artichoke and Spinach Dip

Ingredients

- 1 pkg. Cream Cheese
- 1 can 14 oz. Progresso Artichoke Hearts, drained, coarsely chopped
- 1/2 cup Spinach, frozen chopped, or steamed
- 1/4 cup Mayonnaise (do not use Miracle Whip)
- 1/4 cup Parmesan Cheese
- 1/4 cup Romano Cheese (You can use all Parmesan)
- 1 clove garlic, finely minced
- 1/2 tsp. fresh basil (dry 1 tbsp. Basil)
- 1/4 cup Mozzarella Cheese grated
- 1/4 tsp. Garlic Salt
- Salt and Pepper to taste

Allow cream cheese to come to room temperature. Cream together mayonnaise, Parmesan, Romano cheese, garlic, basil, and garlic salt. Mix well. Add the artichoke hearts and spinach (careful to drain this well) and mix until blended. Store in a container until you are ready to use. Spray pie pan with Pam, pour in dip, and top with cheese. Bake at 350 degrees for 25 minutes or until the top is browned. Serve with cucumber slices, pork rinds, or sliced celery).

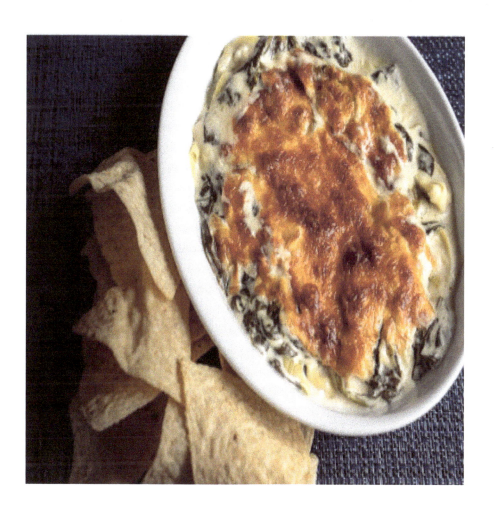

Guacamole Dip or Salad Dressing

Ingredients

- 3 ripe avocados
- 3 Tbsp. lemon juice
- 1 small onion very finely chopped 1 tsp. garlic powder
- 2 Tbsp. mayonnaise Salt and pepper to taste Dash of Tabasco sauce
- Dash of Worcestershire sauce
- Very finely chopped jalapenos peppers to taste
- 1 chopped ripe tomato

Placed peeled and cut avocados in a medium bowl and on low-speed blend with mixer. Add remaining ingredients, adding jalapenos to suit your taste, and blend until the mixture is thoroughly mixed together but not soupy. Chill and serve on lettuce as a salad or with chips as a dip. Place avocado pits in the mix while being stored in the refrigerator to keep the mixture from turning dark.

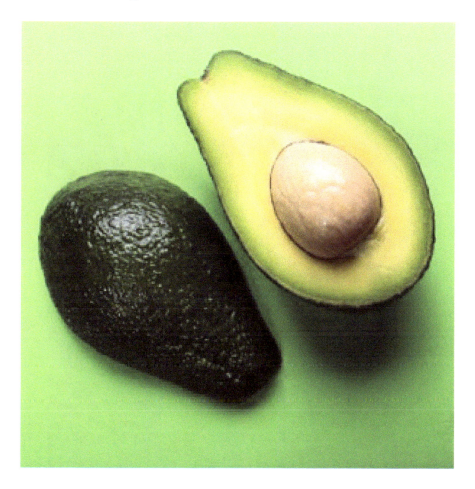

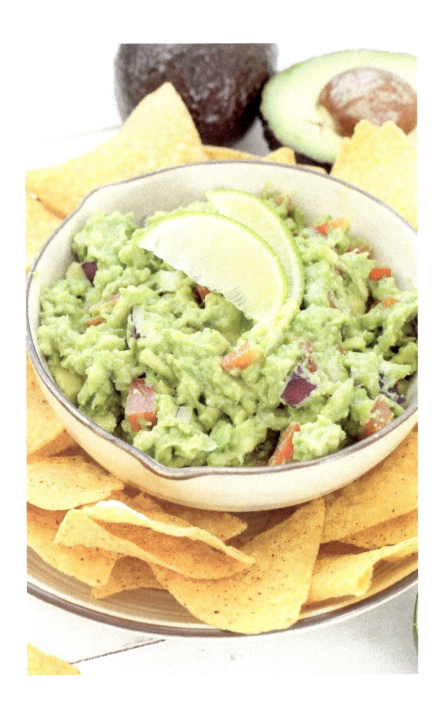

Hot Crab Dip

Ingredients

- 8 ounces cream cheese, softened
- 1 tbsp. cream
- 1 pound lump crab meat use the canned or fresh mixed with the canned
- 2 tbsp. finely chopped onions
- 1 tsp. horseradish
- 1/8 tsp. black pepper
- 1/2 cup toasted almonds

Preheat oven to 375: Combine the cream cheese and milk; add the crabmeat, onion, horseradish, and pepper. Blend well and spoon into an ovenproof dish. Sprinkle with toasted almonds—Bake at 375: for 15 minutes. Serve hot with vegetable sticks or pork rinds as dippers. Serves 8-12.

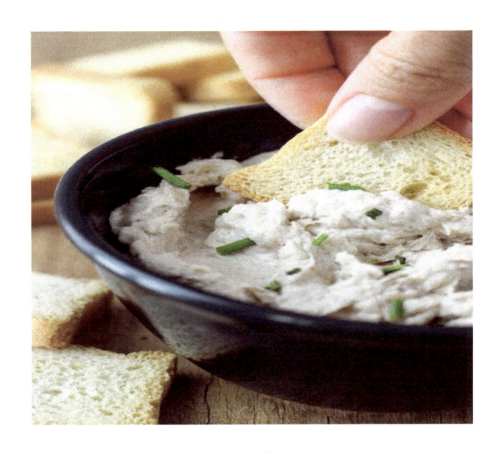

Crab-Cheese Dip

Ingredients

- 2 cans (6 1/2 oz. each) crabmeat
- 1 container (8 oz.) creamed cottage cheese
2 tbsp. mayonnaise
- 1 tbsp. prepared mustard
- 1 tbsp. lemon juice
- 1/2 tsp. salt Parsley
- Twisted lemon slices

Drain crabmeat thoroughly—Reserve the reddest pieces for garnish. Put the remaining half in a container of electric blender with cheese, mayonnaise, mustard, lemon juice, and salt. Whirl until blended. Place in a bowl and garnish with remaining crabmeat, parsley, lemon slices.

Tuna Dip

Ingredients

- 1 six-ounce tin can of tuna
- 1 eight oz. brick of cream cheese warmed to room temperature (or a maybe even little warmer, so that it's really soft)

Mash the cream cheese and the tuna together, put into a nice bowl, and serve with pork rinds, celery sticks, cauliflower, etc.

Chicken Cheese Dip

Ingredients

- 2 cups chopped, cooked chicken
- 3/4 cup mayonnaise
- 2 green onions, minced
- 1/2 tsp. dried basil
- 1/4 tsp. Dried thyme
- 1/2 tsp. salt
- 1/4 tsp. pepper
- 1/2 cup grated Swiss cheese
- 1/2 cup grated Parmesan cheese

Preheat oven to 350°. Mix together chicken, mayonnaise, green onions, spices, Swiss cheese, and 2 tablespoons of Parmesan cheese. Put the mixture in a buttered casserole dish. Sprinkle the rest of the Parmesan cheese on top. Bake about 10 minutes, until the top is browned.

Cheese Puffs

Ingredients

- 1 pkg. (3 oz.) cream cheese (they'd be good with pepper cheese, too)
- 1/4 lb. sharp cheddar cheese
- 1 stick butter
- 2 egg whites, stiffly beaten Pork Rinds

Melt cream cheese, cheddar cheese, and margarine in a double boiler. Fold cheese mixture into stiff egg whites. Dip pork rinds. Let stand in the refrigerator overnight. Bake the puffs in a slow oven, 250 digs., for about an hour, or until crisp. The texture comes out like a cookie.

cream cheese 3 carbohydrates

cheddar cheese 4 carbohydrates

egg whites 6 carbohydrates

Total carbohydrates: 7.6

Store in an airtight container.

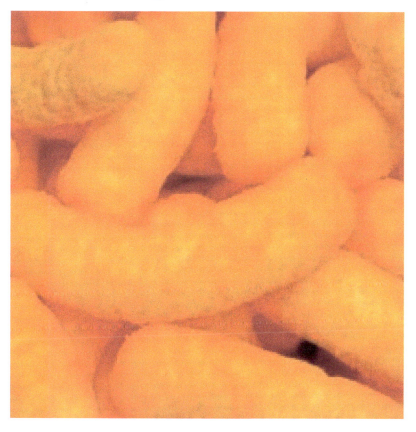

Stuffed Mozzarella

Serving Size: 4

Ingredients

- 4 ounces mozzarella cheese
- 3/4-pound fresh spinach steamed
- 2 red bell peppers sliced lengthwise 1 tablespoon balsamic vinegar
- 2 cups mixed salad greens 2 tomatoes sliced

Flatten fresh mozzarella to 1/2" width—layer with spinach and red peppers. Roll up jellyroll fashion from the longest end. Slice and serve with greens, tomatoes slices drizzled with balsamic vinegar.

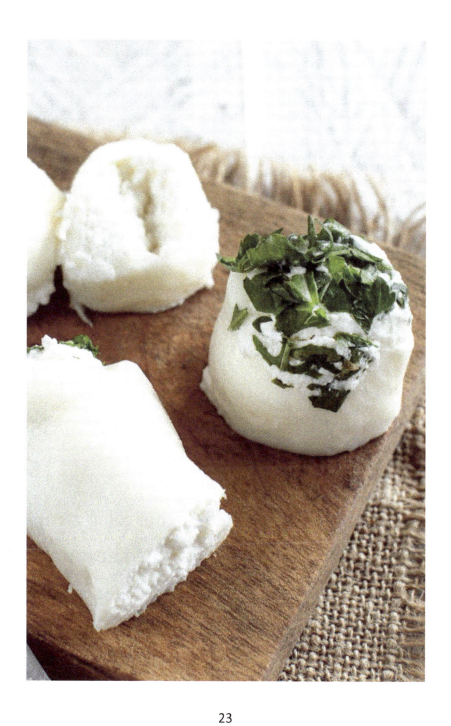

Artichoke-Spinach Dip

Ingredients

- 1 cup chopped artichoke hearts (canned or frozen and thawed) drain the canned ones
- 1/2 cup frozen, chopped spinach, thawed
- 8 ounces cream cheese
- 1/2 cup grated Parmesan cheese
- 1/2 tsp. crushed red pepper flakes
- 1/4 tsp. salt
- 1/8 tsp. garlic powder Dash of black pepper

Boil the spinach and artichoke hearts in a cup of water in a small saucepan over med heat until tender, about 10 minutes. Drain well in a colander. Heat the cream cheese in a small bowl in the microwave set on high for 1 minute. Or use a saucepan to heat the cheese over med heat just until hot. Add the spinach and artichoke hearts to the cream cheese and stir well. Add remaining ingredients to the cream cheese mixture and combine. Serve hot with crackers, chips, etc. Serves 4 as an appetizer.

Fresh Crab Cocktail

Ingredients

- 2 cups tomato sauce
- 2 tablespoons horseradish (fresh if available)
- 2 tablespoons Burgundy wine (optional)
- 1 tablespoon lemon juice
- 1/4 teaspoon pepper
- 1/2 teaspoon salt

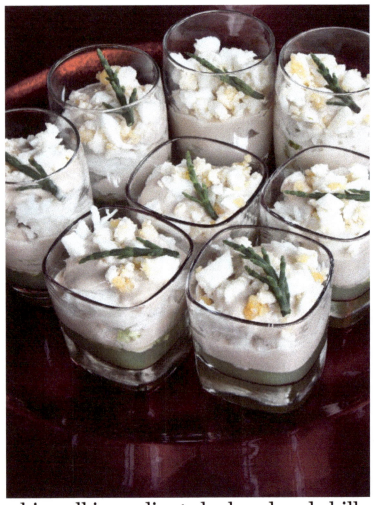

Combine all ingredients by hand and chill thoroughly.

Crab Cocktail

Serves 4

Ingredients

- 2 whole fresh Dungeness crab, cleaned and cracked
- Shredded fresh iceberg lettuce
- 2 fresh lemons, quartered

Line a serving bowl with the shredded lettuce. Arrange a cracked crab attractively on top of lettuce and garnish with lemon quarters. Serve cocktail sauce in a separate bowl.

Crabbie Spread

Ingredients

- 1 stick butter, room temperature
- 1 jar Kraft Old English Cheese Spread
- 1 Tbsp. mayonnaise
- 1 can crab (approximately 7 ounces)
- Minced garlic or garlic powder to taste

It's fabulous briefly broiled or baked at 400 until bubbly and browned, but what to put it on is a bit of a problem on low carb. I tried Wasa crackers, which came out rather soggy and not very good. Portobello mushrooms might work better as a base. Or stuff it in some celery sticks or use rounds of zucchini as a base.

Cheese Ball

Ingredients

- 16 oz. Cream cheese (softened)
- 2-3 green onions (chopped)
- 3/4 tsp. mustard
- 1 tbsp. mayonnaise
- 1/2 tsp. Cayenne pepper 1 tsp. paprika
- 1 tsp. Accent
- 1 tsp. garlic powder
- 1 tsp. Worcestershire sauce
- 1 tsp. Tabasco sauce (optional) 1/2 cup chopped pecans

Mix all ingredients except the pecans, and shape into a ball. Roll the ball in pecans and enjoy!!!

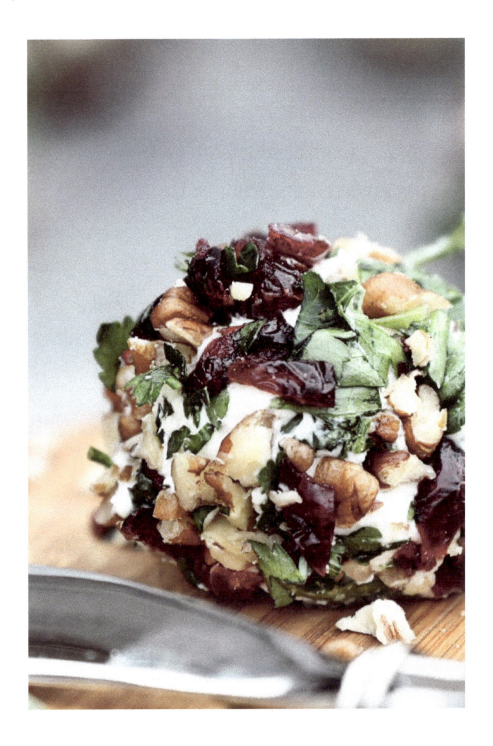

Options for Chips and Dippers

Take one American cheese slice, place or parchment paper or heavy-duty freezer wrap in the microwave, and microwave for 1 minute 10 seconds, until crispy.

Take very thinly sliced cooked salami, place between paper towels, and microwave until crispy! Almost like a potato chip without the potato

Sliced fresh vegetables make good dippers. Try spears of broccoli, slices of mushroom, cucumber, or zucchini, spoons of sweet red and green pepper.

Hollow out cherry tomatoes and fill with any spread or dip.

Any sliced deli meat can be covered with a spread or dip and rolled-up for great finger food.

Cream cheese/Bleu cheese/Pesto

Ingredients

- 1 8 oz brick of cream cheese
- 4 oz crumbled blue cheese or more to taste
Pesto sauce
- Chopped sun-dried tomatoes (preferably in olive oil)

Let the cream cheese come to room temperature. Mix in the blue cheese—Line a small Tupperware container or the like with wax paper. Spread half of the cream/blue mixture in the container. Put a thin layer of pesto, followed by a thin layer of the sun-dried tomatoes. Spread the rest of the cream/bleu cheese mixture in. Cover and refrigerate.

Chicken "Paste"

Ingredients

- 4 boneless chicken breasts
- 16 oz of cream cheese
- 16 oz of sour cream
- One packet of taco seasoning Lettuce
- Cheese (grated)

Take the first four ingredients and combine them in a food processor w/metal blade. This is the basic "paste" or dip. Then make a layer of lettuce and cheese. Fairly simple. Way too much food for two people, we'll be eating it with pork rinds for days, and I'll probably have to eat it for a couple of meals. There are about 10 carbs in a taco seasoning packet, but it is so much food, a serving will make that negligible.

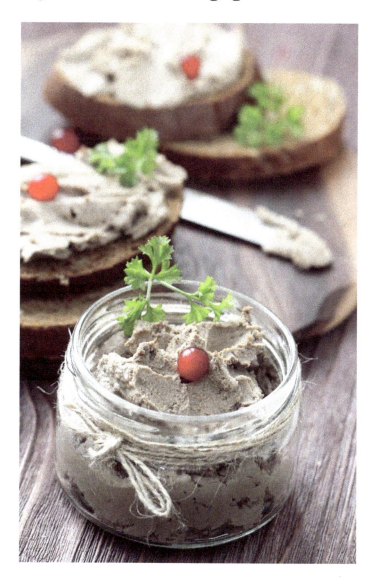

Bacon Cheddar Dip

This concoction is so simple and so tasty, and so versatile you will probably end up using it a lot this coming holiday season

Ingredients

- 16 oz sour cream
- 2 cups shredded cheddar cheese
- 2 oz real bacon bits
- One envelope ranch dressing mix or ranch party dip mix

Combine all ingredients in a bowl, cover, and chill for one hour. It can be used as veggie/pork rind dip, or you can use it over chilled chopped cauliflower for baked faux auto salad.

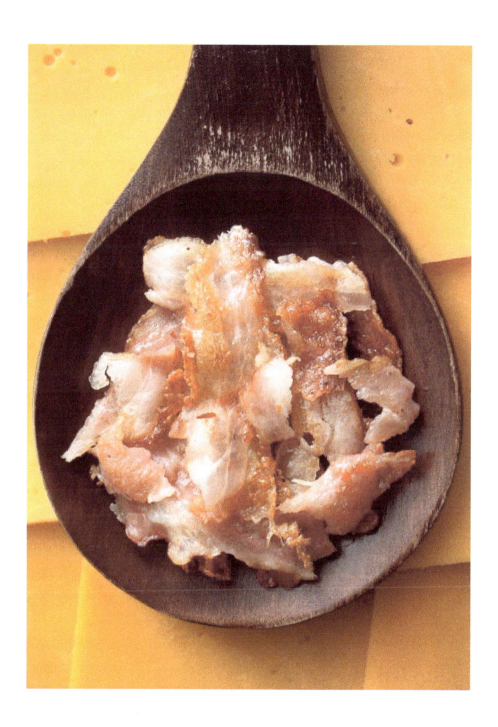

Toasted Seasoned Nuts

Ingredients

- 2 tablespoons butter
- 1 teaspoon seasoned salt
- 1 teaspoon seasoned pepper
- 1/2 teaspoon garlic powder
- 1/2 teaspoon sale
- 1/4 teaspoon cayenne pepper 1 cup whole almonds
- 1 cup pecan halves 1 cup walnut halves

Preheat oven to 300. Melt butter in a large skillet. Stir in spices. Stir in nuts to coat. Pour in a rimmed baking sheet and spread in a single layer—Bake for 10 minutes. Stir and bake 10 minutes longer or until lightly toasted. Cool and store in an airtight container.

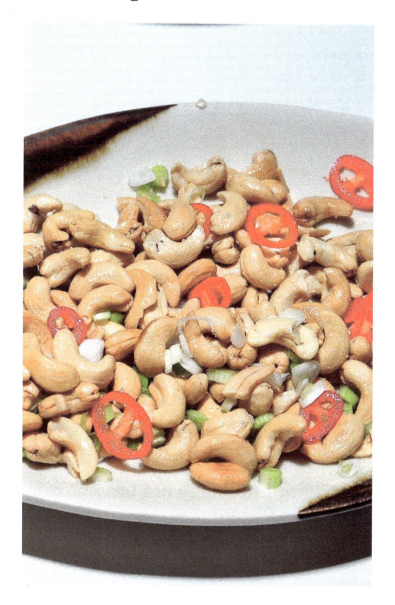

Stuffed Mushrooms

Ingredients

- Whole Mushrooms
- Fresh Cream Cheese
- Packaged Dried Beef

Pull the stems off the mushrooms and use them for something else (I toss them). Chop up the beef - I use about 1/4 package for 8 oz mushrooms. Mix the beef with 4 oz cream cheese. Stuff the mushrooms (a little overflowing) with the cream cheese mixture and bake at 350 until the cheese is a little brown.

You could bring this as an appetizer to a party and then you'll have something to eat too!

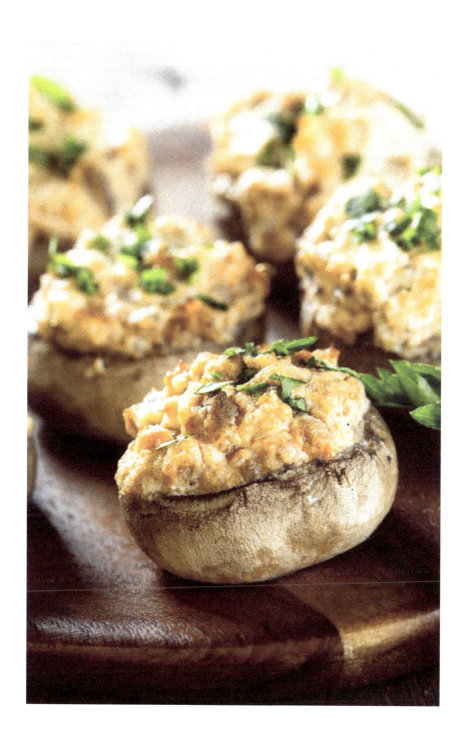

Spinach Dip

Ingredients

- 16 oz Sour cream &/or mayonnaise or combo of both
- 1 -2 pack frozen spinach thawed, drained, and squeezed
- 1 tbsp. garlic powder or 1 clove of minced fresh garlic
- 1 tbsp. oregano
- 2 tbsp. dried parsley or 1/4 c fresh chopped
- 1 bunch chopped green onion
- Salt & pepper
- 1/2 tsp. chili powder

Mix and refrigerate overnight. Add more seasonings to taste.

Guacamole

Ingredients

- 1 med. tomato, peeled
- 2 ripe avocados, black or green
- 3 Tbsp. finely chopped, canned green chilies (I use mild, but you can use whatever you want
- 1/2 cup finely chopped onion
- 1-1/2 Tbsp. White vinegar
- 1/8 tsp. pepper

In a medium bowl, crush tomato with a potato masher

Peel avocados halve crosswise and remove pits. Slice avocados into a crushed tomato. Crush with tomato until well blended

Add chile peppers, onion, vinegar, and pepper. Mix well

Refrigerate, covered, until well chilled--at least 1 hour.

Hope you like it. Holds for about a week. Try it with Grilled chicken slices on top of onions, mushrooms, and green peppers. Add a dollop of sour cream. Also great with pork rinds.

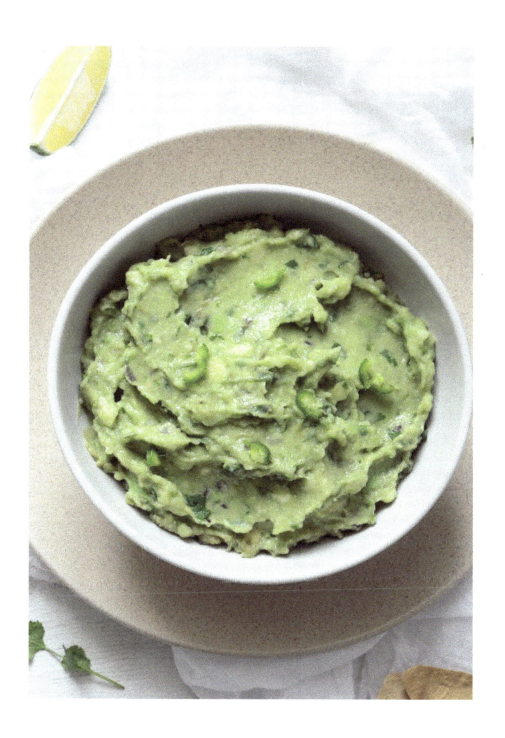

Salsa Cheesecake

Ingredients

- 3 8-ounce packages of cream cheese
- 3 eggs
- ½ cup low-carbohydrate salsa (check the nutritional information on the label)
- ¾ cup sour cream
- ½ cup chopped red pepper
- ½ cup chopped green onion
- ½ cup grated cheddar cheese

Preheat oven to 325. Beat cream cheese with eggs until blended. Mix in salsa. Spray a 9-inch springform pan with cooking spray. Pour cheese/egg/salsa mixture into the pan and bake for 45 minutes. Remove from oven, and cool for

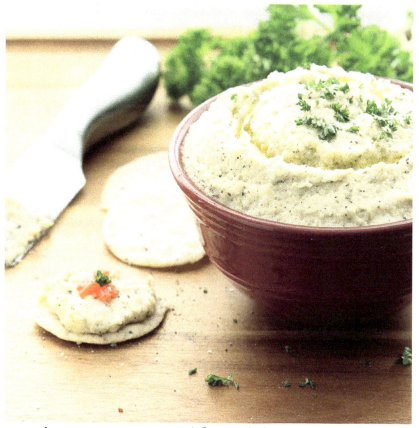

10 minutes. Loosen sides of the pan and cool to room temperature. Remove sides and chill until just before serving.

Spread top of cheesecake with sour cream and sprinkle with red pepper, green onion, and cheddar cheese.

Cut in wedges to serve.

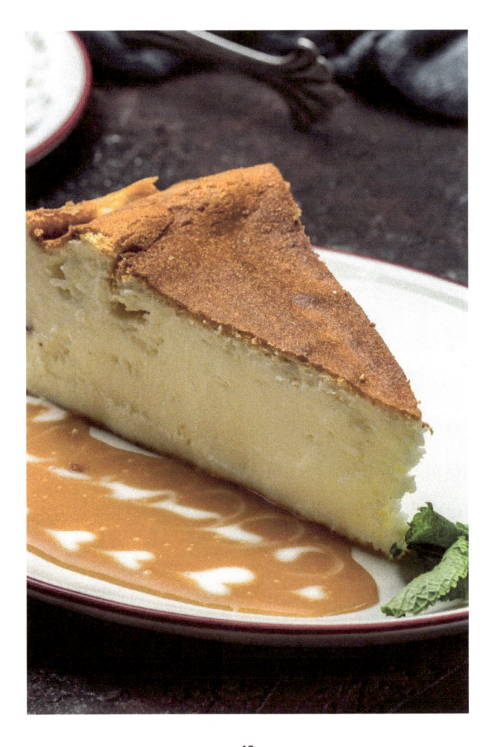

Curried Pumpkin Seeds

Ingredients

- 1/4 cup curry powder
- 1 clove garlic, crushed
- 1/4 cup hot water
- 1 cup of water
- 1 teaspoon salt
- 2 cups plain pumpkin seeds melted butter
- (optional-- cayenne pepper)

Combine the curry powder, garlic, and hot water; mix until blended. Add 1 cup of water and salt. Heat to a simmer, stirring constantly. Add the pumpkin seeds, and simmer for 5 minutes; drain. Spread the seeds on a cookie sheet, brush with a little melted butter and sprinkle with additional salt and perhaps some cayenne pepper. Toast under the broiler until lightly browned. Makes 2 cups.

About 40 seeds equal about 7 carbs.

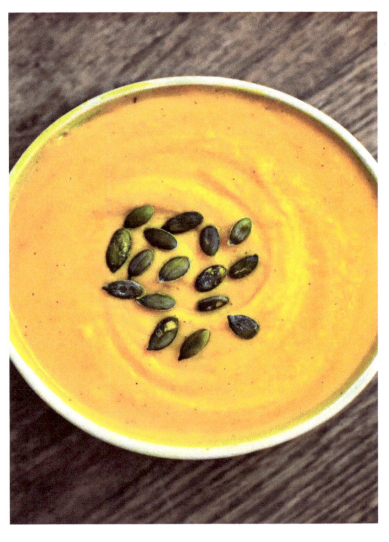

Smoked Gouda-Stuffed Chicken Wrapped in Bacon

Serves Four

Preheat oven to 350

Ingredients

- degrees 4 boneless chicken breasts
- 3 TBS butter
- Salt
- ½ tsp. Black pepper
- ½ tsp. Garlic powder
- ¼ tsp. Paprika
- ¼ tsp. cayenne
- ½ cup smoked Gouda cheese 4 slices bacon

Flatten each chicken breast to ¼ inch thickness. Combine pepper, garlic powder, paprika, and the cayenne together in a small bowl and spread evenly on both sides of the chicken breasts. Salt to taste. Cut the smoked Gouda into small pieces and place one-quarter of the cheese on each breast. Press down firmly and roll the breast, starting with the narrow end. Wrap each chicken breast with one piece of bacon. Melt the butter in a skillet over medium heat. Brown the chicken rolls evenly in the butter until the bacon begins to crisp. Place the four chicken rolls in a baking dish and bake at 350 degrees for 20 minutes.

Serve immediately.

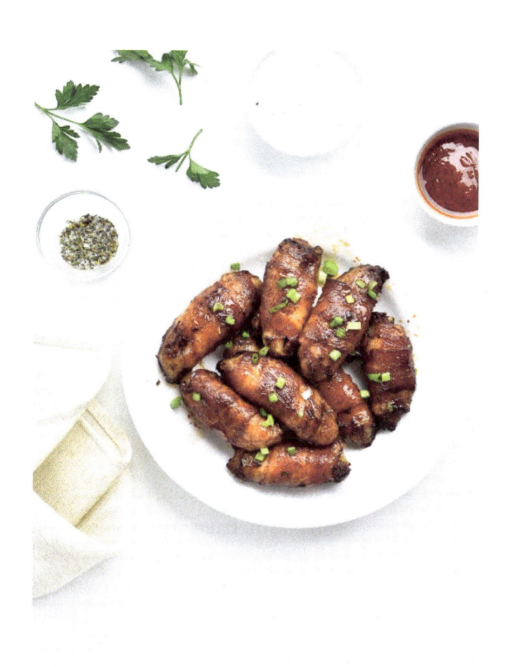

Beef Coin Snacks

Ingredients

- 12 ounces lean minced beef
- 3-4 ounces bacon
- Salt, pepper, garlic powder, dried parsley

Combine a liberal amount of seasonings with meat. Roll up in Saran wrap until it resembles cookie dough. Twist ends. Chill for several hours. Remove and reserve plastic wrap. Cut in half—wrap rolls in bacon. Bake on a rack pan to catch drippings at 375 for 40 minutes. Cool.

Remove bacon, cut bacon in pieces, fry and use in a salad, etc. Rewrap meat rolls and chill well. Slice in ¼ inch rounds. Good for snacking or dipping.

Oysters in Gruyere Sauce

Ingredients

- 24 oysters on the half shell
- 1 tsp. cornstarch
- 3/4 cup heavy cream
- 1 tablespoon unsalted butter
- 1/2 cup plus
- 1/3 cup coarsely shredded Gruyere or swiss cheese
- 1 tbsp. Pernod (anise-flavored liqueur)
- Fresh chervil or parsley for garnish

Heat Broiler. Arrange oysters on a large broiler pan. Whisk cornstarch into the cream in a small saucepan. Add butter and bring to boil, whisking; boil 1 minute. Remove from heat, stir in 1/2 cup cheese, and Pernod until cheese melts. Divide and spoon sauce over oysters; top evenly with remaining 1/3 cup cheese. Broil oysters 4 inches from heat 4 to 6 minutes, until golden.

Low-Carbohydrate Guacamole

Ingredients

- 1/2 avocado
- 1 cup of mayonnaise
- A squeeze of lemon juice
- 2 cloves of garlic
- 1 teaspoon of salt
- 1 teaspoon of chili powder.

YUM! Use cheese "crackers" or celery to dip.

Tapenade

Ingredients

- 1 c. black olives (kalamata suggested)
- 2 drained anchovy fillets (optional)
- 1 tbsp. drained capers
- 2 tbsp. lemon juice
- 1 tbsp. olive oil
- 2 tbsp. brandy
- 1 tsp. Dijon mustard
- 1 tsp. Chopped fresh thyme or 1/4 tsp. dried
- 1/4 tsp. black pepper

Place pitted olives in food processor/blender with remaining ingredients. Blend until finely chopped.

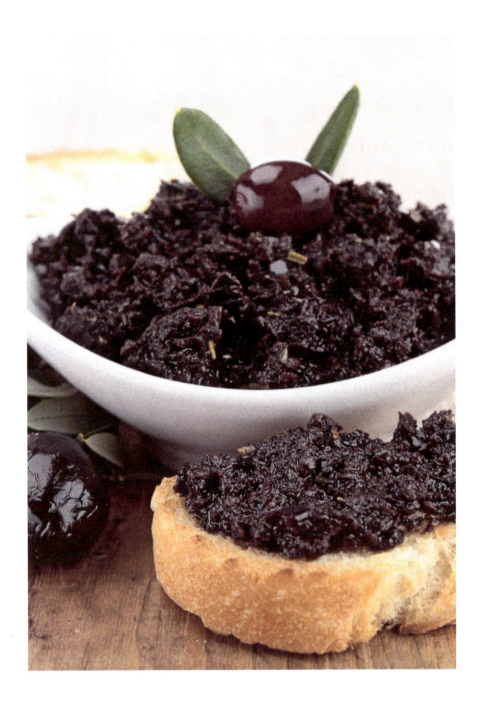

Mozzarella Sticks

Ingredients

- 3 chicken thighs with skin (this left a lot of leftover 'batter' for use on other days. Use less if you like, but make sure to use less of the other ingredients as well.)
- 8 sticks of mozzarella cheese (size is a preference thing; mine were 1 1/2" long and 1/2" around)
- 1/4 cup of crushed pork rinds
- Hot sauce to taste 1 large egg
- 2 tablespoons of Parmesan cheese

Boil the chicken thighs in a pan of water until they are thoroughly cooked. Remove them from the pan and pour the stock into a freeze-able container to use with other recipes later. Remove all the meat from the bones in whatever manner you like. Waiting until they're cool is probably a good idea, but if you have little time, use a knife and fork and cut the meat off.

Get out your blender and grind the chicken into a paste, trying to make sure there are no unground bits left. Somehow get it out of the blender and into a bowl. Add the hot sauce, pork rinds, and egg and mash with a fork until all ingredients are thoroughly blended.

Take a stick of cheese and coat it with some of the 'batters.' It will be VERY sticky, so expect to have messy hands. Try to keep the coating as thin as possible while entirely covering the cheese. Rolling them between your hands helps the 'batter' to hold together better. After you have them coated, roll them in the parmesan cheese so that they're lightly dusted and not sticky to the touch.

When all the sticks have been coated, fry them in a pan of hot oil, turning them often to make sure they don't burn. Once they are crispy golden, you have your delicious Mozzarella Sticks! Enjoy!

Obviously, you can add whatever seasonings to the 'batter' that you like. I'm a hot sauce addict, so that's what I used. You can add Parmesan right to the 'batter' mixture, salt and pepper, whatever! Use your imagination!

Fried Vietnamese Spring Rolls

Ingredients

- 1 lb. ground chicken or pork (uncooked)
- 2 cups shredded cabbage
- 2 cups shredded carrots
- 1 bunch green onions chopped
- 1/2 cup shitake mushrooms, soaked, drained, finely diced
- 1 package small cellophane noodles, soaked, drained, chopped finely
- 2 eggs
- 1 T garlic powder/garlic salt 1 T onion salt
- 1 T pepper
- 1 tsp. salt
- 1 tsp. sugar
- Lumpia wrappers or rice paper.

Mix all ingredients together for filling. If using rice paper, you have to dip them into hot water and lay them on the counter. They will become soft and pliable.

If using lumpia wrappers, keep them covered with a wet paper towel to don't' dry out. Mine is 4g carbs per sheet.

Use won ton wrappers for dumplings or potstickers (mine are 16 grams of carbohydrate for 5 pieces.

For the spring rolls, lay the filling on the bottom third (not middle) and fold up the bottom, then the two sides, and roll up cigar style. For potstickers and dumplings, place filling in the middle and fold up half like moon shape. Pan-fry dumplings till golden brown on each side, then put in a little chicken broth to steam for about 15 minutes.

For low carb filling, I omit the noodles, cut the carrots and onions in half, and omit the sugar. My mother currently makes them with just chicken. She's tired of all that chopping! Food processors do great for shredding carrots and cabbage etc...

Dipping sauce:

Make your own low carb sweet and sour sauce or the traditional Vietnamese dipping sauce: 1 part water

- 1 part sugar
- 1-part white vinegar

Microwave for till sugar dissolves. Add 1-part Asian fish sauce (noun mam) and add hot chili peppers to taste.

This refrigerates till the end of time and can be used as a dipping sauce, marinade, dressing, etc...

You can make gallons or 1 cup. Just use EQUAL PARTS!!!

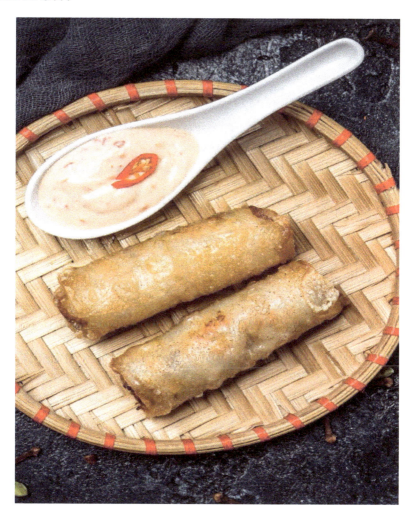

Homemade Antipasto

Crush (or shave with a garlic shaver/grater rather than a press) 4 cloves of garlic and mix with olive oil, vinegar (I used red wine and balsamic vinegar), basil, oregano, pepper, & rosemary. Chop in pepperoni, mild white cheese (I used mozzarella and Havarti). Add olives, quartered, artichoke hearts, and just about anything else you could want. let it steep in the fridge for 2

days and gave it an occasional shake. The only thing with many carbs is the artichoke hearts, but you only eat 2-3 pieces of artichoke (1/2-3/4 of a heart) per serving because it is so pungent and filling. YUM!

Mushroom Pate

Ingredients

- 1 Tbsp. butter
- 1 (8oz.) package chopped mushrooms
- 1 oz chopped Portabello mushroom
- 1/4 cup crumbled blue cheese
- 2 tbsp. dry sherry

In a large frying pan, melt butter over high heat; add mushrooms. Cook, often stirring, 4 minutes or until mushrooms begin to brown and liquid is gone. Sprinkle with blue cheese; stir in sherry. Continue cooking until cheese is melted.

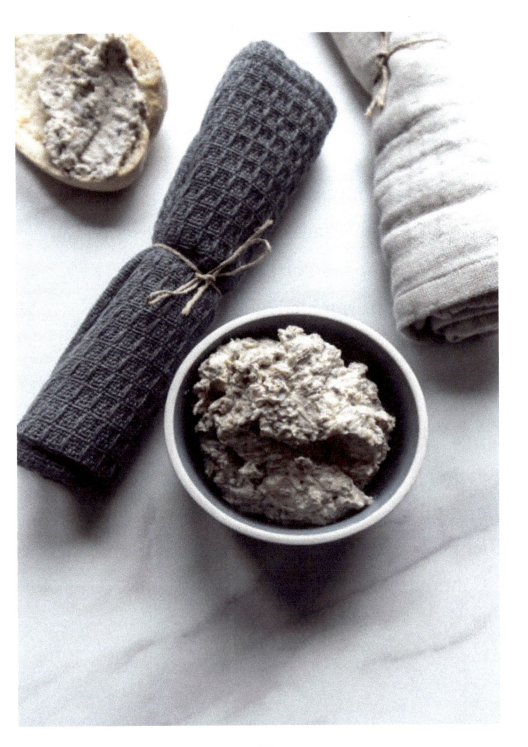

Crab Stuffed Mushrooms

Ingredients

- 7-10 oz crab meat (I used crab leg meat, chopped in a food processor)
- 5- Scallions- chopped fine
- 1/4 tsp. Thyme & Oregano
- Black Pepper to taste
- 1/3 cup mayo
- 1/2 cup grated Romano cheese

Preheat oven to 350. Remove stems & gills from mushrooms to make a small cup. Combine all other ingredients. Chill. Stuff the mushrooms sprinkle w/grated Romano & paprika. Bake for 15 minutes. Serve w/ Lemon wedges.

Pickled Shrimp

Serves 12 to 15 as an hors d'oeuvre

This popular cocktail party dish never fails to please a crowd, and there is never any leftover.

The fact that it should be made at least a day in advance is a big bonus when planning a party, and the proportions can be increased to serve any number of guests.

Remember to go easy on the salt when increasing the recipe.

Ingredients

- 3 pounds shelled and cooked shrimp
- 3 onions, sliced very thin
- 7 or 8 bay leaves
- 1 1/4 cups salad oil
- 1/4 cup white vinegar

- 1/2 tablespoon salt
- 2 1/2 teaspoons celery seeds
- 2 1/2 tablespoons undrained capers
- Generous dash of Tabasco Pepper Sauce
- 1 garlic clove crushed

Make alternating layers of shrimp and onions in a shallow glass dish. Combine remaining ingredients and pour over shrimp. Cover and refrigerate for 24 hours or longer. Drain off marinade and serve icy cold in a bowl (in a large shell looks excellent) with a small toothpicks container to spear the shrimp.

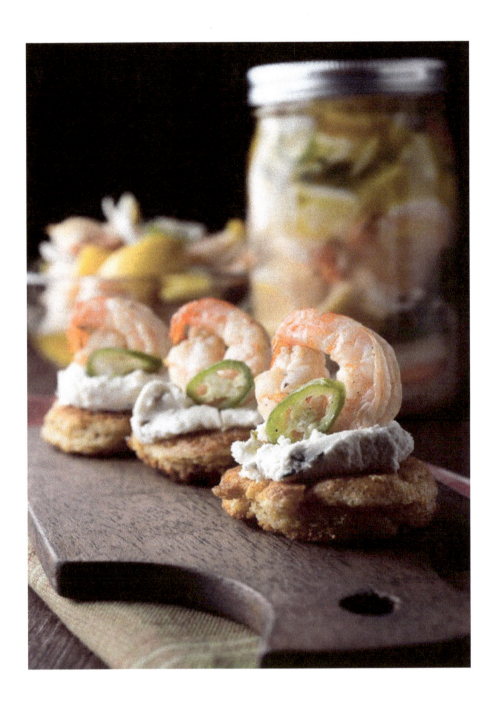

Crabmeat Dip

This makes a double batch. I used to eat this on crackers, but now I enjoy it from cokes to pork rinds.

Ingredients

- 4 cans crabmeat (drained)
- 2 small chopped onions
- 1 cup mayonnaise (or more if needed to make it creamy)
- garlic powder to taste
- Parmesan cheese
- Paprika

Mix the first four ingredients and place in a casserole dish. Sprinkle Parmesan cheese on top to cover and sprinkle a little paprika on that. Bake at 350 degrees for 15 minutes or until bubbling at edges.

Salmon Dip

Ingredients

- 1 8oz cream cheese
- 1 tbsp. Horseradish or Worcestershire sauce Chives (lots or little your choice)
- 1 small can of pink salmon, drained
- Anice little shot of Lemon juice
- A drop or two of red food coloring (to make it all pinkish)

Once the cream cheese is softened, mix all ingredients together, as desired.

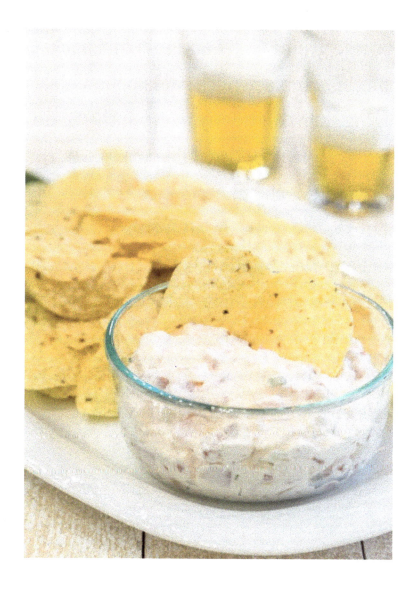

Carbohydrate-free Nachos

Cook some ground beef and toss in a package of taco mix. Then place pork rinds on a plate, arranging them optimally to catch the "fixin's," but the taco meat all over the pork rinds, then the shredded nacho cheese, next to the jalapenos. Now nuke for about 1 minute or until cheese is melted. Wallah!!! Not too bad. Not bad at all. The seasoned meat helps you forget the refried beans. And you don't have to use jalapenos if you don't like em that hot. Or you can toss on Tabasco or low carb salsa.

Spinach Dip

Ingredients

- 1 box frozen chopped spinach
- 3 tablespoons grated Parmesan cheese
- 3 tablespoons low-carb ranch dressing
- 1/2 cup sour cream
- 1/2 tsp. Dried basil 1/2 tsp. garlic powder

Thaw spinach. Combine all ingredients in a bowl; mix well. Serve chilled

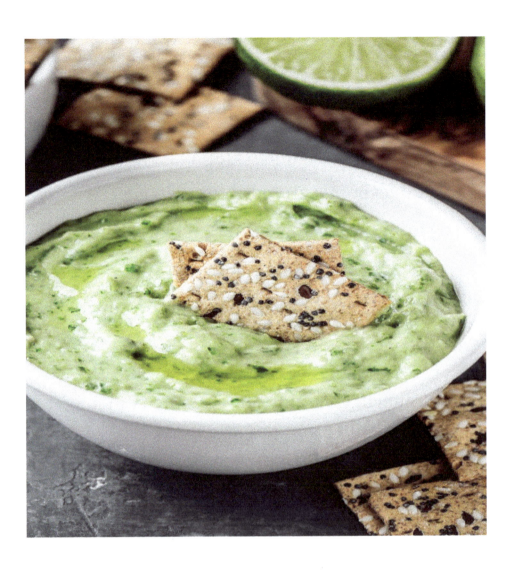

Hot Crab Dip

Ingredients

- 1 pound (16 ounces) Maryland backfin or jumbo lump crabmeat
- 1 package (8 ounces) cream cheese, softened
- 1/2 cup sour cream
- 2 tablespoons mayonnaise
- 1 tablespoon lemon juice
- 1-1/4 teaspoons Worcestershire sauce
- 1/2 teaspoon dry mustard 1 tablespoon milk
- 1/4 cup cheddar cheese, grated
- Pinch garlic salt, paprika for garnish

Carefully pick through crabmeat, removing any shell pieces. In a large bowl, mix cream cheese, sour cream, mayonnaise, lemon juice, Worcestershire sauce, mustard, and garlic salt until smooth. Add enough milk to make the mixture creamy. Stir in 2 tablespoons of grated cheese. Fold crabmeat into cream cheese mixture.

Portobellos with Feta and Artichokes

Brush 4 large mushroom caps with liquid from artichoke marinade and broil on both sides, 2 minutes on each. Chop artichoke hearts and add 1/2 cup crumbled feta and 1 small tomato diced. Place mushrooms on a plate, ribbed side up, and put 1/4 of the mixture on each. This is a great first course.

Scallops or Shrimp with Bacon

Marinate sea scallops cut in half or large deveined shrimp in your favorite dressing or teriyaki for a few hours or overnight. Take skewers and put one end of a slice of bacon on, then a piece of seafood, bring bacon over and onto a skewer, and repeat till you have 6 shrimp or scallops on ending with bacon. Grill or broil until bacon is cooked. 2 per person for an entree or one for the first course.

Low-Carb Cheese sticks

I cut small square strips of mozzarella, dipped them in egg and rolled them in crushed pork rinds (plain or hot n spicy), and set them in a nonstick pan with some hot oil for a few seconds, and flipped them until they were done, and they were great.

Thai Shrimp Dip

Ingredients

- 1-pound medium shrimp, cooked and peeled
- 1/4 cup (2 ounces) cream cheese
- 2 tablespoons mayonnaise
- 2 tablespoons fresh lime juice
- 2 teaspoons Thai fish sauce or low-sodium soy sauce
- 1 (12.3-ounce) package firm tofu, drained
- 1 teaspoon dark sesame oil
- 1 tablespoon minced peeled fresh ginger
- 1 garlic clove, minced
- 3 tablespoons minced green onions
- 3 tablespoons chopped fresh cilantro
- Cooked and peeled shrimp (optional)
- Cilantro sprig (optional)

Place the first 3 ingredients in a food processor and process until minced. Add lime juice, fish sauce, and tofu, pulse until blended. Heat oil in a small skillet over medium heat; sauté ginger and garlic for 2 minutes. Add to shrimp mixture, and pulse until combined. Add onions and chopped cilantro, and pulse 3 to 4 times. Spoon into a bowl; cover and chill for 1 hour. Garnish dip with additional shrimp and cilantro sprig, if desired.

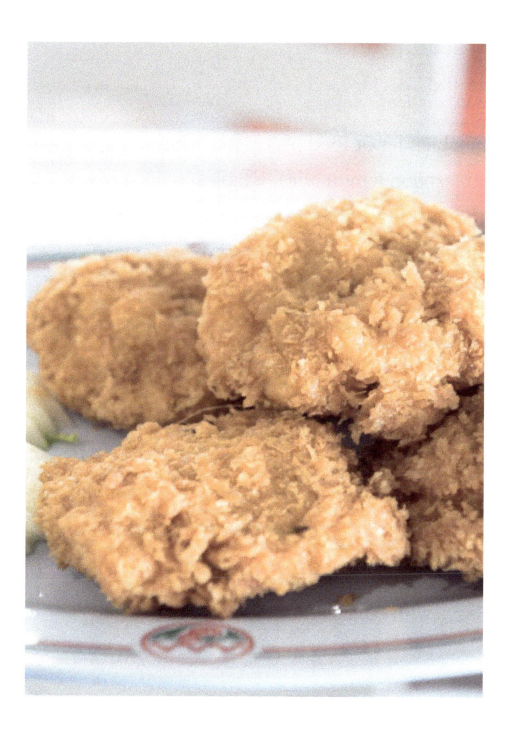

Macadamia Pesto

In a blender or food processor, whirl 1 tablespoon lemon juice, 3 tablespoons olive oil, and 1/4 cup salted, roasted macadamia nuts until coarsely ground. Add 3 tablespoons of grated parmesan cheese and 11/2 cups lightly packed rinsed and drained fresh basil leaves. Whirl until smooth, scraping container sides as needed. Add salt to taste. Makes about 1/2 cup.

Per tablespoon: 90 cal., 88% (79 cal.) from fat; 1.7 g protein; 8.8 g fat (1.5 g sat.); 1.8 g carbs (0.9 g fiber); 54 mg sodium; 1.5 mg cholesterol. Serve with (suggestions from the group)

*   We use pesto on spaghetti squash all the time. It's also great on shrimp, chicken breast meat, and grilled veggies.

*   Add some garlic to the pesto when you make it, then slather on top of chargrilled red/yellow/orange capsicums or any other grilled vegetables. Add to chicken salad with mayonnaise and cheese. Anoint a hot grilled steak, even on top of a cheese omelet. Also, try mixing with cream cheese and filling celery sticks.

BEVERAGES

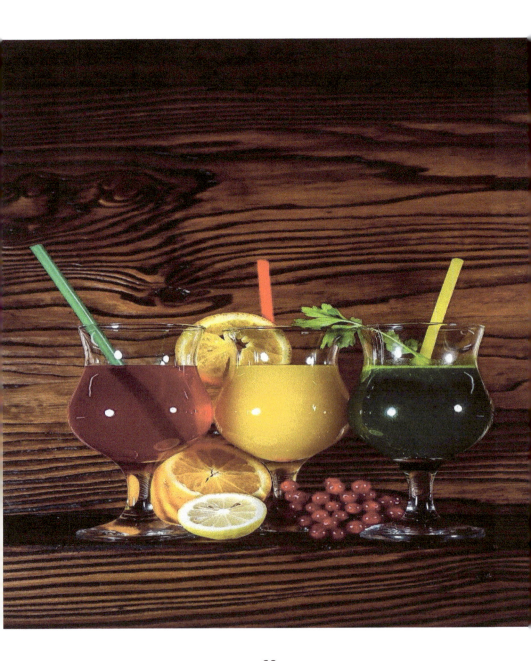

Chocolate Shake

Ingredients

Put in blender:

- 1/4 cup cream
- 1/4 cup cottage cheese
- 1/4 cup egg substitute
- 1/2 cup water
- 1 Tbsp. cocoa
- 1 heaping Tbsp. Equal or Splenda
- 2 heaping Tbsp. low carb protein powder (optional)

Blend a few minutes, then blend in about 8 cubes of ice, one at a time.

Hot Chocolate

Ingredients

- 1 tsp. cocoa powder
- 2 tsp. Splenda
- 8 oz hot water.
- 1 tsp. instant coffee

Mix together and enjoy!

Frappuccino

Brew 4 cups strong coffee. (make expresso if you like. I use a French press for a full extraction) Add 1 cup to 1.5 cups cream

15 to 30 drops of liquid sweet n low

Stir then cool. Store in fridge, pour over ice and enjoy.

....

Strawberry Shake

Ingredients

- 1/2 C Land O'Lakes gourmet whipping cream
- 2 T Equal
- 1/2 C Strawberries
- 1/4 C water
- 5 ice cubes

Blend in blender until ice is integrated into the mixture. Serve.

Protein Shake

Ingredients

- 2 Standard Scoops Protein Powder 2 Tbsp. Canola or Flax Seed Oil
- 1 tsp. Sugar-Free Laxative 1/2 tsp. Vanilla (optional)
- Cinnamon to taste (optional) water

In a shaker bottle, mix powders. Then add oil & shake well until oil is completely absorbed by powders. Fill to top with water and shake well. Allow standing at least ten minutes. Shake again & drink. The laxative will expand as it stands, giving the drink a creamy texture. Very low-carb.

Protein "Milkshakes"

Ingredients

- Use flavored Protein powder: vanilla, chocolate, banana, plain.
- 1 to 2 scoops of vanilla egg protein powder (24 g pro. & 1 g = carb. each)
- 1/3 cup cream (about 2 g carb.)
- 2/3 c water
- 1/3 c frozen strawberries (4.5 g carb).

Whirr is a blender till combined.

Quick Protein Shake

8 oz unsweetened soy milk (5g carbs, 4g fiber) ***This is not the same as "plain" soy milk.

Make sure it's sugar-free!***

Ingredients

- 4 oz heavy cream (1.65g carbs)
- 1 scoop sugar-free vanilla protein powder (1g carbs)
- Some sugar-free DaVinci vanilla syrup (0g carbs) (I guess I use about 3 tbsp.)
- 1/2 tsp. sugar-free Tang (0g carbs)
- 4-5 cubes of ice

In the blender, till it's smooth -- delicious!

Hot Cocoa

Ingredients

- 1/4 cup heavy cream
- 3/4 cup boiling water
- 1 tbsp. cocoa powder Sweetener to taste

Mix the cream with cocoa powder until dissolved. Add boiling water and sweetener (I use about 10 tablets). Mix until sweetener has dissolved, and enjoy!

Coconutty Protein Shake

Ingredients

1/2 cup unsweetened coconut milk

1/4 cup Healthy N Fit 0-carb egg protein powder (vanilla flavor, but all the ingredients read is "vanilla flavoring" - no sweetener)

1/2 cup water 3-4 ice cubes

1/2 tsp. vanilla (or other extract depending on the flavor of shake)

2 rounded tsp. sugar-free instant pudding powder, the flavor of choice Sweetener to taste, if desired

Combine all ingredients except ice cubes in a blender and blend until mixed. Add ice cubes and blend for a couple more minutes. Pour into a glass and enjoy.

Shake Shake

Here is a shake I used to use after my workouts in the gym or football field. I still use it now on my Atkins/PP hybrid diet. Tastes good and good for you.

Ingredients

- 1 scoop chocolate Designer Protein (whey protein)
- 1 scoop of N-R-G protein powder (soy, casein, whey, egg proteins) 1 whole egg
- 2 tablespoons macadamia nut oil (mmm mmm good)
- 2 packets of Equal
- 1/2 cup of half and half 2 cups of water
- 4-5 ice cubes

I find this shake a treat and use it as a dessert most of the time. Most other shakes I have to force down. Hope this helps you out some.

Protein Shake ala Light

Ingredients

- 1 1/2 cups Crystal Light any flavor (already mixed with water)
- 4 tablespoons heavy whipping cream
- 2 scoops carb-free, fat-free vanilla egg protein powder
- 1-ounce cream cheese
- About 1 cup of ice cubes

Whip and enjoy. A Pitcher of this lasts me all day, sometimes 2, depending—about 5 carbs.

Favorite Protein Shake Recipe

Ingredients

- 12 oz very cold diet orange soda
- 2 scoops vanilla flavored protein powder, preferably Jay Robb
- 2 oz cream
- 1 cup or so of ice

Combine above in blender, blend for 1 1/2 minutes, pour, and serve. The cream can be omitted if dairy sensitive.

Tastes fabulous.

Protein Power Shake

Ingredients

- 1/2 cup raspberries, sliced strawberries or peaches,
- fresh or frozen 1/2 cup cottage cheese
- 1/4 cup plain yogurt

Crystal Light or Sugar-Free Tang (already mixed, not the powder) to taste, enough to cover all the other ingredients in the blender jar.

Mix in the blender. You can add ice if using fresh fruit.

The Frugal Gazette Diet Drink

Ingredients

- 7 Tbsp. powdered egg white
- 4 Tbsp. regular flavor, smooth texture Metamucil with no sugar or sweeteners
- 20 packets diet sweetener (I suppose you could use sugar to taste if you are watching out for fat and not for carbs)
- 1 c. and 2 Tbsp. non-fat dry milk for flavor
- 4 Tbsp. Powdered unsweetened cocoa 6 tsp. vanilla extract
- 1 package powdered unsweetened drink mix ("Kool Aid"), strawberry or raspberry

Dry mix: place egg whites, Metamucil, sweetener, and dry milk into a bowl.

Thoroughly mix all ingredients. Add the desired flavoring and store it in a sealed container at room temperature. (If using vanilla extract, stir until evenly distributed and allow to dry in an open container for 2-4 hrs)

To Reconstitute Drink Mix: Add 3 Tbsp. of dry drink mix to 1 ½ cups cold 1% or skim milk. For best results, use a blender, food processor or shake vigorously in a closed container.

Protein Shake Base with Variations

(about 28g protein, 5g carb)

Ingredients

- 1/2 cup cottage cheese (rinsed in a strainer, if it has a sour taste)
- 1/2 cup pasteurized egg whites (Second Nature Eggs, has no onion or garlic-like Egg Beaters do)

For each variation, add the following ingredients and whirr in a blender

Variation 1 Peach Melba

- 4 oz. (by weight) frozen sliced unsweetened peaches (about 6g carb)
- Dash of DaVinci SF raspberry syrup
- 2 or 3 packets of sweetener
- 1 cup of water

Dash of cream optional

Variation 2 - Berry Shake

Ingredients

- 1/3 cup frozen unsweetened blueberries or 4 oz frozen unsweetened strawberries (about 6g carb) 2 or 3 packets sweetener
- Dash of vanilla extract (about 1/2 tsp) 1 cup water
- Dash of cream optional

Variation 3 - Chocolate Shake

Ingredients

- 1 tsp. Chocolate extract, or 1 heaping tsp. cocoa 2 or 3 packets sweetener
- Dash of vanilla extract (about 1/2 tsp.) Dash of cream (few Tbsp.)
- 1/2 cup water 6 ice cubes

Shake Recipe

Ingredients

- 1/4 cup heavy cream
- 1/4 cup water
- 1/4 cup pasteurized egg substitute, like "EggBeaters."
- 1/4 cup cottage cheese: I strongly recommend Breakstone's or Knudsen's
- 1 tablespoon protein powder, any type
- 1/2 teaspoon good-quality sugar-free vanilla extract 6 Equal tablets, crushed
- 1 cup crushed ice (about 7 ice cubes)

Blend all ingredients at high speed until no visible pieces of ice or cottage cheese remain. This makes a vanilla shake containing roughly

330 calories, 5 carbs, 21 grams of protein, and 25 grams of fat. For a bigger shake, use 1/3 cup of each egg sub, cheese, water, and cream instead of 1/4 cup each, add 3 more ice cubes, 3 more Equal tablets, and a teaspoon more protein powder. The larger shake contains about 450 calories, 7 carbs, 34 grams of fat, and 28 grams of protein.

"Spice Tea" Mix

Ingredients

- 1/2 little tub of crystal light plain iced tea granules 1 tub of the lemon aid flavor
- 1 package of sugar-free orange Jello

Mix all together. Make hot water in a coffee cup like for Tea. Add ½ teaspoon of this mixture and stir till well mixed...add more or less depending on how strong you like it.

Breakfast on the Go

Ingredients

- 1 cup of coffee
- 2 Necta sweet tabs (saccharine equalling 2 tsp. sugar) "correct" amount of half & half for the coffee
- 1 scoop designer protein chocolate flavor
- 5 or 6 ice cubes.

Blend away. Thick, but you can drink it through a straw.

Raspberry Protein Shake

2 scoops of vanilla whey protein (GNC brand or Designer Protein)

Ingredients

- Raspberry syrup to taste
- 1/2 cup water 1/2 cup ice
- 1 oz syrup
- 1 tsp. psyllium powder (for fiber)
- 10 drops liquid stevia

Put in a blender and mix until ice is crushed.

Hot Chocolate

Ingredients

- 1/2 cup cream
- 2/3 cup water
- 1 tsp. unsweetened cocoa
- 1 packet sugar substitute
- 1/2 tsp. vanilla

Place all ingredients in a saucepan. Heat to the boiling point, but do not boil. Stir constantly. Serve in a mug. Total carbohydrate grams: 5.4.

"Bailey's and Coffee"

Ingredients

- 1 cup hot decaffeinated coffee (this is usually prepared at night. no caffeine then)
- 1 tbsp. Heavy cream 1 tbsp. Jack Daniels
- 1 tsp. Splenda (or to taste)

It is soooo good!!

Eggnog

Ingredients

- 1/2 cup plus 2 tbsp. Splenda
- 2 eggs, separated

- 1/4 tsp. salt
- 2 cups heavy cream 2 cups water
- 1 tsp. vanilla
- Brandy or rum flavoring to taste
- 1/2 cup whipping cream,
- whipped Ground nutmeg, or cinnamon

Beat 1/2 cup Splenda with egg yolks. Add salt, stir in 2 cups cream and water. Cook over medium heat, continually stirring, until the mixture coats a spoon. Remove from heat and allow to cool. Beat egg whites until foamy, then gradually add remaining Splenda, beating to soft peaks. Add to the cooked mixture and blend thoroughly. Add vanilla and flavoring. Chill for at least 3-4 hours. Pour into punch bowl or cups—dot with "islands" of whipped cream. Sprinkle with nutmeg or cinnamon.

Egg Not

Ingredients

- 2 cups Skim milk
- 2 packages substitute sweetener
- 2 tsp. vanilla extract
- 1/4 tsp. rum extract
- 1/2 cup egg substitute (thawed if frozen)
- 1 tsp. nutmeg

Combine milk, sweetener, vanilla, and rum extract. Beat with egg substitute until well blended. Chill and stir before serving.

1 serving: Carbs (w/milk) 10 grams.

Lightning Source UK Ltd.
Milton Keynes UK
UKHW021914190221
378991UK00005B/57